AI in Fitness Tracking

Modern Tools for Healthier Lifestyles

Table of Contents

Chapter 1. Introduction

In this eye-opening Special Report, we delve into the exciting intersection where artificial intelligence meets fitness tracking, powering innovations that are transforming our approaches to health and wellness. This isn't just about counting steps or calories anymore, it's about harnessing complex technology to foster healthier lifestyles — yet, we've gone the extra mile to make this report highly accessible, even if you're not tech-savvy. You don't need to be a computer scientist or a fitness guru to appreciate these modern tools, which are putting more potent, personalized health strategies right at our fingertips. With this report, understand the cutting-edge world of AI in fitness tracking and how it's inspiring us to make leaps, not just steps, on our path to improved health. So, let's get fit smarter, not harder!

Chapter 2. Unfolding the Importance of Fitness Tracking

In the grand scheme of personal health, fitness tracking has not only evolved to become a noteworthy trend but a critical tool for individuals pursuing a healthier lifestyle. The surge in the importance of fitness tracking is attributed to the increased accessibility of personalized biometric data, enabling us to understand how our bodies respond to different types of physical activities, diets, and lifestyle changes.

2.1. Understanding The Explosion in Fitness Tracking

In the earliest stages of fitness tracking, pedometers were utilized to simply count the number of steps walked within a day. But the landscape of fitness tracking has expanded tremendously. With modern advancements in technology, fitness trackers can measure everything from heart rate to sleep patterns to blood oxygen levels. As a result, monitoring personal health has grown more intuitive, sophisticated, and proactive, marking a shift from consultation and treatment to real-time tracking and prevention.

Fitness trackers, most commonly found in the form of wearable devices and mobile apps, are now considered critical components of fitness regimens. They present users with a wealth of information that provides context to not only their workout routines but also their overall wellbeing. By allowing individuals to make more informed decisions pertaining to their health and fitness, trackers inspire users to maintain a consistent, healthy lifestyle.

2.2. Delving Deeper into Fitness Tracking

The evolution of fitness tracking has empowered us to access personalized health data more than ever before. This data is often presented via engaging and user-friendly metrics, charts, or outcomes, making wellness tracking far more than an activity—it's a lifestyle. Each detail helps generate a comprehensive picture of a user's health, fostering personal investment in their fitness journey.

For instance, a running app not only tracks the distance and time of your runs but can also take note of your routes, pacing, elevation changes, and even how your performance varies under different weather conditions. Similarly, sleep tracking apps offer insights into your sleep cycles—highlighting any irregularities or disruptions—to ensure optimal rest and recovery.

2.3. The Shift to Proactive Health Management

This ongoing access to personalized health data has marked a considerable shift in health-related attitudes and practices. People are now better equipped to play an active role in managing their health and wellbeing. With fitness tracking technology by our sides, we can be proactive rather than reactive when it comes to taking care of our bodies.

Health, in its holistic sense, is no longer viewed through the narrow lens of dieting or exercising alone. Instead, it encompasses a blend of the physical, emotional, and mental states harmoniously working together. Accordingly, fitness tracking devices now offer insight into stress management, recovery times, sleep quality, nutrition intake, and more, reflecting a 360-degree view of health.

2.4. Fostering Healthier Habits

Fitness tracking plays an important role in habit formation, too. Visualizing physical activities, health markers, and the progress made overtime can act as a powerful motivator. It's human nature to crave palpable progress, and this tracking provides exactly that. Many fitness tracking apps utilize tactics like weekly reports, challenges, badges, or social sharing features to keep users engaged and reinvigorate their drive for better health goals.

These tactics not only encourage more regular physical exercise but they also incentivize lifestyle adjustments, such as prioritizing sleep or managing stress. Over time, these small changes acquire the status of healthy habits, forming the backbone of a healthy lifestyle full of vitality and vigor.

2.5. A Foundation for Personalized Fitness

Possessing detailed biometric data and tracking health patterns enables an unparalleled level of personalization in the world of fitness and health care. Fitness tracking devices can learn from our behaviors, adjust to our routines, and predict our needs. They can recommend workouts, customize plans, and even adjust daily goals based on how you've been eating, moving, or sleeping.

In essence, through fitness tracking, each person's fitness journey becomes unique, tailored, and personal, making the approach to health not only strategic but also manageable and sustainable. It's about making the world of fitness work for you, rather than trying to keep pace with an unrealistic, one-size-fits-all approach.

In conclusion, the importance of fitness tracking cannot be understated. It's a transformative tool in personal health and wellness that fosters awareness, encourages healthier habits, and facilitates personalized strategies for optimal health. As technology continues to evolve, so too will fitness tracking, paving the way for even more profound insights into our health and wellbeing. Understanding this only motivates us to cherish and utilize this technology, making the fitness journey a part of our lifestyle and not just a leisure activity. The ultimate objective of fitness tracking, after all, is to allow us to live our healthiest, best lives—by leaps and bounds!

Chapter 3. Decoding Artificial Intelligence: A Simplified Introduction

Artificial intelligence, often abbreviated as AI, is increasingly becoming a buzzword, not only in tech circles but also in everyday life. It is driving change in various sectors, from healthcare to transportation, and even fitness – a realm we'll be exploring further in this report. Let's start by simplifying what AI is.

AI refers to the simulation of human intelligence in machines, programmed to think like humans and mimic their actions. It's about creating smart machines capable of problem-solving, learning, adapting, and performing cognitive tasks. Essentially, AI is a broad area of computer science that makes machines seem like they have human intelligence.

3.1. Understanding the Types of AI

To better comprehend AI, let's dissect it into three types:

Simplified AI: This is the most basic and widely-used AI type. Simplified AI systems are created to perform tasks such as voice recognition, recommendation systems, or search algorithms but are incapable of learning or adapting.

Limited Memory AI: This type of AI can learn from historical data and improve over time, but it's limited to the specific task it was designed for. A quintessential example would be self-driving cars that collect data from their sensors to learn about the world around them.

Self-learning AI: This is the most advanced type of AI, which not only learns from historical data but is also capable of conscious thought or self-awareness. However, this type of AI currently exists more in theory than in practice.

3.2. AI in Action: Examples

There are many examples where AI has been integrated into our everyday lives:

1. Virtual Personal Assistants like Siri and Alexa are AI technologies that recognize natural language and respond to voice commands.

2. Artificially intelligent algorithms power navigation apps like Waze or Google Maps, getting us from point A to point B efficiently.

3. In music or video streaming services, AI is used to analyze your preferences and suggest songs or shows accordingly.

3.3. The Science Behind AI

Now that we have a basic understanding of what AI is and its different types, let's delve into the science behind it. AI incorporates various techniques and algorithms to function effectively. A few fundamental elements include:

Machine Learning (ML): ML is a subset of AI. It's a system that can learn from data, identify patterns, and make decisions with minimal human intervention.

Neural Networks: These are algorithms inspired by human brain function and designed to imitate its behavior. They are complex patterns of code that can process data in an incredibly sophisticated manner.

Deep Learning: This is a subfield of machine learning, which makes the computation of multi-layer neural networks feasible. It essentially teaches computers to do what comes naturally to humans: learn by example.

Every one of these elements has a wealth of information within them, and we've only scratched the surface. They represent the intricate, fascinating science that forms the cornerstone of AI.

3.4. The Intersection of AI and Fitness

In recent years, AI has been making waves in the fitness industry, triggering an evolution from simple step-counting to creating personalized workout and diet plans based on user's individual health data.

AI-powered fitness apps use algorithms to analyze your workout data and make fitness recommendations tuned to your needs. This transformation not only offers information about your physical activity but also brings insights about the quality of your workouts, current fitness level, and potential health risks.

Now that we've decoded the reality of AI, in the next chapters, we'll dive deeper into understanding how these technological advancements intersect beautifully with fitness tracking — redefining our approach to health and wellness.

Let's remember, understanding AI doesn't require extensive technical knowledge. With a basic concept in mind and an open attitude, we can better appreciate how this technology is transforming our lives. The aim is to discover how to utilize AI's potential to our benefit and work smarter towards our fitness goals — not harder.

Chapter 4. AI and Fitness Tracking: A Marriage of Tech and Health

In recent years, we've seen the rise of an interesting tech-health union leveraging Artificial Intelligence (AI) in fitness tracking. This potent combination not only improves our physical well-being but also revolutionizes our understanding and approach towards overall health. Let's dive in and explore the digital revolution redefining how to get fit and healthy.

4.1. Understanding AI and Fitness Tracking

In essence, AI is the technology that enables machines to learn and adapt through experience, simulating human-like intelligence. On the other side of the marriage, fitness tracking is the process of monitoring and recording physical activity levels, as well as other relevant health data.

Initially, fitness tracking was straightforward and manual—the daily task of writing down meal descriptions, counting steps or calories burned. With advancements in technology, however, fitness tracking devices were developed that could automatically and electronically collect and analyze these data, making tracking more efficient and accurate.

The introduction of AI into fitness tracking technologies has been a game-changer. Imagine having a personal trainer who understands your body like a scientific researcher, tracks your progress like an obsessed fan, and tailors your fitness plans with exceptional precision. This is what AI makes possible in fitness tracking.

4.2. The Rise of AI in Fitness Tracking

AI-powered devices use algorithms to understand, learn, and predict user behavior and performance, enabling them to provide personalized and proactive recommendations. These instruments can monitor heart rate, sleep patterns, activity levels, and offer personalized workouts.

In the past few years, there has been an explosion of innovative products and apps powered by AI. These include wearables, smart sport equipment, AI-powered coaching apps, and more. At its core, each innovation exhibits a deepened emphasis on consolidation, personalization, and gamification driven by AI.

4.3. The Mechanics of AI in Fitness Tracking

AI in fitness tracking operates primarily on data gathered by sensors embedded in devices such as wearable fitness trackers, smartphones, and sports equipment. This data consists of raw numbers representing heart rate, distance traveled, calories consumed, and more. With machine learning, a subtype of AI, these raw numbers are interpreted and used to make useful recommendations for the user.

Machine learning algorithms need to be trained using large datasets to make accurate predictions. The more data, the more nuanced the algorithm's understanding, leading to more accurate and personalized advice on fitness routines, diet plans, or activity levels.

4.4. Personalized Coaching with AI

AI provides a degree of personalization and adaptation that is nearly impossible for humans to achieve. For example, using the data gathered from a user's activity levels, sleep patterns, and heart rate, an AI algorithm can create a tailored workout plan that best fits that individual's fitness goal and current state.

The AI can adapt the program as the user progresses or if their goals change, making it like a digital personal coach. The use of AI here mitigates the one-size-fits-all approach to fitness planning and makes fitness journeys more personalized, motivating and effective.

4.5. AI and Adaptive Fitness Programs

The potential of AI in fitness isn't limited to monitoring and personalized coaching alone. AI-powered adaptive fitness programs are now a reality. From customized yoga sessions to strength training routines, AI has been changing the landscape of fitness training.

These adaptive programs work completely on the user's conditions. It's efficient and smart—it adapts to your level, adjusts to your schedule, recovers with you, and constantly challenges you. The idea is that no two workouts need ever be the same, and it should always feel like it is tailored for you.

4.6. Gamification: Making Fitness Fun

Coupled with AI's ability to personalize workout routines, the rise of gamification in fitness tech has made the previously daunting task of exercise more engaging and fun.

Gamification integrates game-like elements into fitness routines. Challenges, rewards, and community achievements are all part and parcel of this approach to improve motivation. AI improves this system through personalized and adaptive challenges based on the user's performance data, ensuring the user is always motivated, challenged, and engaged.

4.7. The Future of AI in Fitness Tracking

With advancements in technology and the proliferation of data, we are likely to see even better AI-powered fitness tracking tools. Predictive analytics, genomics and biometric data combined with AI may yield products and apps that not only lead to better workouts but will also provide broader health benefits.

While much progress has been made, there remains an immense untapped potential in the intersection of AI and fitness tracking. As these technologies continue to evolve and interface, they promise to generate radical new ways to guide us on our journeys towards better health and fitness.

However, like any new technology, privacy and data security issues are paramount. These issues become even more critical when dealing with personal health and fitness data. Therefore, it is essential that thorough security measures are put in place to protect user data and ensure that this promising marriage of technology and health continues to flourish safely.

To conclude, the marriage of AI and fitness tracking brings a revolution to health and fitness management. It allows for personalized, adaptive, and gamified fitness journeys in ways we couldn't have envisaged a few years ago. This technological revolution isn't just counting steps—it's taking giant leaps towards fostering healthier lifestyles. Thus, let us celebrate this union, embrace the benefits, and jump on the bandwagon to achieve our fitness goals. After all, the future of fitness is not just about working harder—it's about working smarter, powered by AI.

Chapter 5. The Mechanics of AI-Assisted Fitness Trackers

Fitness tracking is not a new phenomenon. For years, we've been wearing devices that count steps, estimate calories burned, or measure heart rate. However, with advancements in artificial intelligence (AI), these devices are becoming increasingly intelligent, accurate, and personalized. In recent years, AI has revolutionized many sectors, and fitness is no different. AI assisted fitness trackers provide a deeper understanding of our bodies and health, analyzing complex data and providing actionable insights to optimally reach our fitness goals.

5.1. Understanding Artificial Intelligence

AI is a vast field of computer science that involves the creation of systems which can perform tasks that would normally require human intelligence. These tasks include learning from experiences, understanding complex content, recognizing patterns, data analysis, and decision-making. For fitness trackers, AI takes in vast amounts of data, analyzes it, and spews out actionable insights personalized for each individual.

Machine learning, a subset of AI, plays a crucial role here. It allows fitness trackers to learn from the user's behavior and adapt its responses accordingly. This learning makes the device smarter over time—helping users understand their bodies better and make informed decisions about their fitness and health.

5.2. The Role of AI in Fitness Trackers

AI assists fitness trackers in several ways, contributing directly to their accuracy, effectiveness, and customization.

Predictive analysis is one such application. By analyzing past data, fitness trackers can predict future behavior, helping users keep track of their progress and adjust their fitness plans accordingly. For example, if a tracker notices that a user consistently does not meet their daily step count on Tuesdays, it might suggest additional walking during lunch break or after work times on that specific day.

AI also enables biometric data collection. This includes heart rate, skin temperature, oxygen levels, and sleep patterns—all crucial factors for assessing one's health and fitness levels. Biometric data contributes to comprehensive health monitoring, enabling preventive care, and early detection of potential health issues.

Personalized training plans are yet another application. Based on users' performance, fitness goals, and physical conditions, AI can create customized workouts, optimizing exercise plans for better results. It's similar to having a personal trainer who knows your strengths, weaknesses, and goals, and continuously updates your regimen based on this knowledge.

Lastly, AI allows fitness trackers to motivate users towards better health habits. It uses gamification elements to make the fitness journey fun, engaging, and ultimately rewarding. Challenges, in-app rewards, and social sharing are all strategies employed by fitness apps to keep users motivated.

5.3. The Inner Workings of an AI-Assisted Fitness Tracker

The functionality of an AI-assisted fitness tracker largely depends on sensors, AI algorithms, and data synchronization. Here's a deeper dive into the inner workings of these trackers.

Sensors embedded in the tracker collect raw data on a variety of metrics. This can range from basic metrics such as steps walked and calories burned to more advanced metrics like blood oxygen level and REM sleep. This data is continuously collected and stored for further analysis.

Next, the collected data is analyzed using AI and machine learning algorithms. These algorithms sift through the collected data, identifying patterns, and drawing correlations. They transform raw data into valuable insight, such as sleep quality assessment, or potential health risks.

Lastly, the processed information is then synchronized across devices. It's presented to you on your smartphone or computer in an easily digestible manner. It could be a score indicating your sleep quality, a warning sign about possible health risks, or a personalized exercise plan.

5.4. Future of AI in Fitness Tracking

The future of AI-assisted fitness tracking looks promising. We can expect even smarter devices, more precise measurements, and more personalized insights in the coming years.

One area ripe for innovation is emotion recognition. AI could potentially recognize emotional states and how they relate to physical well-being. Another exciting area is the integration of AI fitness trackers into healthcare services. The large pool of personal health data collected by AI fitness trackers could be a game-changer for the healthcare industry as it can significantly improve disease prediction, as well as personalized healthcare.

In addition to improvements on existing models, there will be countless new forms of AI-integrated fitness devices in the future. Devices that monitor your nutrition, guide you through workouts, or even clothes that correct your posture—these aren't just ideas for sci-fi novels. With AI, they might become a reality sooner than we think.

Overall, AI-assisted fitness trackers are transforming the way we understand and approach our health and fitness. From counting steps, we've moved to comprehensive health monitoring, personalized training plans, and preventive healthcare. With AI advancements, this revolutionary journey is only expected to accelerate, taking us leaps ahead on our path to improved health.

Chapter 6. Pioneering AI Innovations in Fitness Tracking

The fusion of artificial intelligence with wearable technology has given birth to a new era in health and fitness, one marked by an advanced level of personalization, convenience, and above all, effectiveness. Through AI, our wristbands, heart rate monitors, and other fitness-tracking gadgets have evolved into personal wellness consultants of sorts, constantly learning from our actions and patterns to deliver insights that are tailored to our needs and goals.

6.1. A Revolution in Data Collection & Assessment

Traditionally, fitness tracking has been a rather manual, laborious process. Individuals had to manually count their steps, note down exercise routines, and manually calculate calorie intake. This approach, while certainly better than doing nothing, lacked in speed, convenience, and accuracy.

The integration of AI into fitness tracking has facilitated far better data collection and assessment. Machine learning algorithms are used to analyze movements and detect activities, estimating the number of steps walked, calories burned, and even the quality of your sleep. These algorithms constantly learn from the user's activities and feedback, improving their estimations over time to provide a more accurate assessment of the individual's fitness levels.

These AI-enabled trackers also collect and analyze health data. Unlike their predecessors, they can monitor a range of physiological parameters – heart rate, body temperature, even oxygen levels – and identify abnormal patterns that might indicate potential health issues. The data collected is real-time, which is great because it means you always have an up-to-date picture of your overall health.

6.2. Unveiling the Power of Predictive Analytics

Predictive analytics takes the capabilities of AI in fitness tracking a notch higher. It's not just about understanding what happened in the past or what is happening now; it's about predicting what might happen in the future. Using complex algorithms, AI-run fitness trackers analyze historical and current data, identify patterns, and predict future outcomes.

This feature is quite remarkable. It can, for instance, notify a user when their current rate of calorie intake and exercise would likely lead to weight gain. If someone has had consistently high heart rates during workouts, the AI might predict potential heart health concerns and recommend seeking medical advice.

For runners, predictive analytics could provide an understanding of when they might hit their personal bests or when they're at risk for an injury. The anticipatory capabilities don't just give a new dimension to personal fitness, they create a framework for preventive healthcare.

6.3. Personalized Training, Anytime, Anywhere

Artificial intelligence has been pivotal in making training more personal. By considering an individual's capabilities, goals, preferences, and constraints, AI can generate a workout schedule that is unique to that user. This level of customization goes beyond just varying the type of exercise or durations – the AI differs in how it motivates, instructs, and gives feedback to different users based on their personality types.

Advanced AI fitness platforms feature virtual personal trainers. These are voice-activated AI models, capable of providing audio guidance during workouts. They correct form, recommend alternative exercises,even monitor pacing during a run. By combining real-time feedback with meticulously crafted workout structures, these AI coaches provide the benefits of a personal trainer, right on a user's wrist.

What's more, these AI coaches are always available, function irrespective of location, and don't charge extra for their time. This has opened up personal training to a broader demographic, making professional guidance accessible to those who previously found it too expensive or restrictive.

6.4. Bridging the Mind-Body Gap

Mental wellness has been an often overlooked aspect of fitness. However, progress in AI-based fitness tracking is fostering a more holistic approach to wellness, encompassing both physical and mental health.

Wearable technology is employing AI to evaluate psychological state using indicators like stress levels, sleep quality, and even social media usage. Many wearables now include meditation and mindfulness practices within their catalog of features, often providing personalised endorsement based on the user's emotional state — calculated from the collected data.

Ingesting physical and mental health parameters alongside information about an individual's goals and lifestyle, allows AI to deliver unified and sustainable health strategies. Such inclusivity of mental wellness represents a significant leap forward in our understanding and practice of fitness.

6.5. Conclusion

As impressive as these AI-driven innovations in fitness tracking are, it is clear that we are only at the dawn of what is possible. As technology continues to advance and our understanding of the human body and mind deepens, AI's role in personal fitness is sure to become ever more central.

The key driving factor behind the success of these AI innovations is the ongoing learning process. With constantly improving algorithms, collection of better data, and increasing ability to personalize experiences, AI is set to continually retransform the fitness landscape in the coming years.

These developments are not bringing about a pervasive 'Big Brother', but rather a 'Big Mother', gently nudging, guiding and helping us in making smarter health choices. As we become routine users of these technologies, we grow more attuned to our bodies and minds, leading to greater health awareness and a more proactive attitude towards fitness.

Chapter 7. Personalizing Exercise: How AI Creates Unique Fitness Regimes

Every individual is unique. From the genetic level up to our lifestyles, habits, and physical constitutions, no two people are identical, and as such, fitness regimes need to reflect this essential truth. Enter artificial intelligence (AI), which is revolutionizing fitness and health technology by overhauling the one-size-fits-all approach to physical fitness and replacing it with highly personalized, nuanced fitness regimes.

7.1. The Power of Data in Personalizing Fitness

AI thrives on data, and lots of it. Every heartbeat registered, every step taken, every hour of sleep logged can serve as data points which AI can learn from. Fitness trackers and smart devices automatically log these and so much more, tracking our physical activities, our heart rates, sleep cycles, and our diet often in real-time. Each piece of data reveals a bit more about our health and fitness status.

Collecting data is just the first part of the process. The real magic happens when this data is analyzed. AI algorithms utilize machine learning techniques to find patterns, trends, and correlations within this massive pool of information. The algorithms can then make predictions and suggestions based on these analyses, taking into account previous outcomes and constantly adjusting the model to optimize for better results.

7.2. From General to Specific: AI's Role in Personalizing Workouts

Most current fitness regimes rely on broad guidelines, age brackets, and general health assessments to formulate fitness plans. AI, however, uses the collected data to create a bespoke fitness regime – serving the user with a highly tailored and adaptive workout plan that evolves in synchronization with the user's progress and changing fitness level.

For instance, an AI-driven fitness tracker can adjust your fitness plan based on your recent activities. If you've been surpassing your step goals, your AI might suggest incrementally increasing your target to challenge you further. Conversely, if work schedules are causing disruption in your workout routine, the AI could recommend shorter, high-intensity exercises that would maximize your gains in a tough week.

7.3. Nutritional Control: AI's Part in a Balanced Diet

Balancing dietary requirements with physical activities is the cornerstone of any effective fitness regime. AI helps by tracking not just what, but also when and how we eat. AI can analyze data on consumed quantities of proteins, carbohydrates, and fat and balance these with a person's activity level to provide pertinent nutritional advice.

One can input their meals into tracking apps, detailing the ingredients and quantity. The AI can then offer a caloric breakdown and make suggestions based on your fitness goals. Whether it's putting on muscle mass, losing weight, or just staying healthy, your AI companion can guide you on achieving those through tailored nutritional advice.

7.4. Sleep Optimization: Enhancing Recovery for Better Fitness

Sleep plays an integral part in any fitness regime. Not only is it a central element in recovery, but it also has impacts on performance, mood, and motivation. Wearable devices track sleep patterns, number of hours, and the quality of sleep, all data that are invaluable in understanding one's overall fitness. An AI leveraging this detailed sleep data can suggest changes to bedtime routines, sleeping environments, or even advise on the best time to work out depending on the individual's sleep pattern.

7.5. Personalized Motivation: AI as Your Personal Cheerleader

Even the most effective fitness regime is of no use if it's not followed consistently. Here, AI can act as a personal motivator, drawing upon the data to craft motivational messages, reminders, suggestions or even set up challenges that play into the user's competitive streak. These can all serve as powerful motivation triggers that ensure consistency and progress.

AI's ability to personalize extends beyond workouts and nutrition—it delivers a unique user experience attuned to personal circumstances and fitness goals. AI can not only remind us to get our shoes on and start working out, but it also has the knowledge and ability to adapt and become a more symptom-specific coach, aiding those recovering from surgeries or living with chronic conditions.

7.6. Embracing the Future of Fitness

AI may be a complex piece of technology, but its potential benefits to fitness and health are straightforward. By personalizing fitness regimes to suit individual progression, nutrition, and sleep patterns, AI provides a holistic approach to attain better health.

The personalization brought about by AI in fitness is more than just customization—it's about a revolution in how we approach fitness and health. Humanity's relationship with fitness is evolving in tandem with technology. Harnessing the power of AI and data, fitness is becoming less about general guidelines and more about personalized strategies that reflect our uniqueness. In a world with AI-driven fitness, we are empowered to push our boundaries and make strides towards our personal health goals. Through constant learning and adaptation, AI brings an intelligent edge to our fitness journeys, enabling everyone to exercise smarter, not harder.

Chapter 8. Understanding Data Privacy and Security in AI Fitness Trackers

With the ongoing technological advancements, the fitness and health industry has seen a tremendous evolution. AI fitness trackers have developed from pedometer-like devices into sophisticated systems that gather and analyze a plethora of personal health data. Undeniably, this has brought considerable improvements to our ability to monitor our health and wellness. Still, it's also crucial to acknowledge the concerns revolving around data privacy and security.

8.1. What Data do Fitness Trackers Collect?

Fitness trackers record a staggering variety of information that extends beyond merely steps or distance logged. Most devices collect the following types of data:

- Personal Identifiers: Basic information such as name, age, gender, and contact information.

- Biometric data: This includes heart rate, skin temperature, oxygen levels, sleep patterns, and even stress signals.

- Physical Information: Height, weight, body mass index (BMI), and sometimes specifics like body fat percentage.

- Location data: Many trackers use GPS technology for route tracking during outdoor workouts.

- Fitness data: Steps, miles, calories burned, and other exercise stats.

All this data, when analyzed collectively, can provide unique insights into an individual's health and wellness state and guide personalized fitness strategies.

8.2. How AI Fitness Trackers Store and Use Data

Here's a glimpse into the practices AI fitness trackers generally follow to store and process data:

- Most fitness trackers send data to the accompanying smartphone app via Bluetooth.

- The app computes and organizes the received data for the user.

- Generally, the data is simultaneously uploaded to the company's servers in encrypted format for more detailed analysis.

- AI algorithms often use this server-stored data to discover patterns, draw correlations, predict future outcomes, and offer personalized workout or lifestyle recommendations.

- Apart from device-specific analysis, some companies anonymize and pool data from all users to carry out lifestyle or health trend research.

8.3. Importance of Data Security in AI Fitness Trackers

While the health insights derived from AI fitness trackers help steer users towards healthier habits, this large amount of sensitive data needs top-notch protection.

- Personal Identifiers: Unauthorized access to these pieces of information could lead to identity theft or misuse.

- Biometric Data: Given its sensitive nature, it can be exploited if fallen into wrong hands. For instance, it can be used to infer a person's medical condition or other personal characteristics.

- Location Data: Real-time location data could be misused for stalking or other malicious activities.

So, a breach could have serious consequences not only for privacy but also for the user's safety. Therefore, it's essential that these devices have a strong security framework in place.

8.4. Current Data Security Measures Taken by AI Fitness Tracker Companies

AI fitness tracker companies are aware of these concerns and have set up several safeguards:

- Data Encryption: Most AI fitness trackers use secure Bluetooth connections to transmit data and apply end-to-end encryption when storing or transferring it.

- Anonymous Data: Individual data is often anonymized before it's used for broad research or analysis purposes.

- Regular Updates: Regular software updates are issued to fix any security loopholes and keep the system safe from the latest threats.

- Two-Factor Authentication: Some offer two-factor authentication for additional account security.

8.5. How to Enhance the Security of Your AI Fitness Tracker

As end-users, there are several strategies we can adopt to further shield our data:

- Regular Updates: Always update your device and its accompanying apps to the latest version.

- Secure Connection: Only sync your fitness tracker with trusted and secure connections.

- Privacy Settings: Regularly review your device and app's privacy settings.

- Strong Password: Use a complex and unique password for your fitness tracker account.

8.6. Understanding and Negotiating User Agreements

Remember that user agreements often dictate how the companies can use your data. Hence, it's critical to read and understand these terms:

- Data Collection: Understand what data your device collects.

- Data Use: Know how it uses and processes this data, both for you and more broadly.

- Sharing Policies: Be aware of how and with whom this data could be shared.

- Opt-out provisions: Know your rights if you don't agree with the terms.

A strong understanding of data privacy and security measures can help users enjoy the benefits of AI fitness trackers while side-stepping potential privacy pitfalls. As these devices continue to evolve, recognizing and addressing these concerns become critical to ensuring a pleasant and secure fitness tracking experience.

Chapter 9. Case Studies: Success Stories of AI in Fitness Tracking

Artificial intelligence has immense potential in reshaping the fitness landscape. The integration of AI with fitness tracking devices has opened avenues for personalized training modules, accurate analytics, likelihood predictions, and achievable goal settings, to name a few. To better understand the impact of AI in fitness tracking, we explore some successful case studies in this field.

9.1. WHOOP: Personalizing Fitness with AI

WHOOP is an AI-driven fitness tracking device capturing data 24/7 to provide personalized workout guidance. The wearable technology utilizes AI algorithms to analyze data on heart rate variability, resting heart rate, and sleep performance. With these parameters, WHOOP provides actionable feedback to users for optimal training and recovery.

In one noteworthy case, a user engaged in excessive workouts found she was unable to reach her desired fitness levels despite rigorous routines. Using WHOOP's sleep tracking and recovery score, she realized her body wasn't getting adequate rest to recover from the exacting workouts. After adjusting her sleep patterns and workout intensity as advised by the WHOOP system, she noted significant improvements in her overall fitness.

9.2. MyFitnessPal: Tailored Nutrition with AI

Nutrition plays a critical role in fitness, and MyFitnessPal, a comprehensive diet and exercise app, utilizes AI in a novel way. MyFitnessPal's AI analyzes user-inputted data, gauging eating habits, and nutritional intake, and offers nutrition advice and diet plans tailored to users' unique needs and goals.

A user struggling to lose weight, despite regular workouts, turned to MyFitnessPal. By analyzing his food logs and leveraging its AI capabilities, the app recognized an overconsumption of carbohydrates as the hurdle. The app suggested a revised daily calorie intake and recommended a diet plan with fewer carbs and more proteins. Following this personalized advice, the user soon started shedding weight more effectively.

9.3. Fitbod: Revolutionizing Weight Training with AI

Fitbod, an AI-based app focused on weight lifting and strength workouts, employs AI-powered algorithms to adjust training regimens based on user performance and bodily responses. The algorithm takes muscle recovery into account and suggests optimum workouts on given days.

A user story illustrates Fitbod's effectiveness. The user, new to lifting weights, had seen limited progress with generic workout routines. Using Fitbod, the user received tailored strength-training routines, learning which muscles to target and how intensely. The personalized regimen improved his strength two-fold within a few months.

9.4. Gixo: Group Fitness and AI

In the world of group fitness, Gixo stands out by leveraging AI. Gixo offers live and on-demand fitness classes with the special feature of real-time corrective feedback. By analyzing user-inputted data in real time, Gixo can refine instructions on the fly to ensure users exercise correctly and safely.

One user who previously felt disconnected in large, physical group workout classes turned to Gixo. The app's personalized real-time corrections helped her perfect her postures and enhanced her group fitness experience, proving efficiency is possible even with larger fitness groups.

9.5. Peloton: AI, the New Personal Trainer

Peloton brings AI to home workouts for cycling enthusiasts. Measurements such as speed, resistance, and output power are recorded for each workout and employed for adaptive resistance adjustments, class recommendations, and even real-time competition with other users.

A Peloton user described how the machine's AI gave her the benefits of a personal trainer at a fraction of the cost. The personalized recommendations and adaptive resistance catered to her fitness level and helped her steadily advance her fitness journey, highlighting the power of AI in mimicking personal trainers.

In conclusion, the integration of AI into fitness tracking has already shown impressive results, making health and wellness guidance accessible to all. The case studies presented herein illustrate just the beginning of what AI can do to revolutionize the fitness industry in the years to come. As technology advances, users can look forward to even more innovative and personalized health strategies.

Chapter 10. The Future Predictions: AI and Fitness Tracking

As technology advances, the exciting intersection of artificial intelligence (AI) and fitness tracking is constantly evolving. Witnessing this convergence, we're able to envisage a future of highly personalized and efficient approaches to health and wellness, fulfilling the promise of AI to transform what we thought was possible.

10.1. The Emergence of Personalized Training

Picture this - you wake up in the morning and your smartwatch has already planned your workout for the day, meticulously considering your sleep pattern, caloric intake, heart rate, body temperature, and more. Not only that, but it tracks your progress throughout the session, adjusting the intensity of your workout on the fly based on your performance.

From generic training routines, fitness technology is evolving towards more personalized training sessions. AI-driven fitness applications, using deep learning and pattern recognition algorithms, can analyze and interpret data from various fitness wearables. They can determine exactly what kind of workout your body needs, optimally adjusting the intensity and duration for maximum benefit and minimal risk of injury.

10.2. Evolution of Health Prediction Models

Health risk prediction models have traditionally been plagued by a lack of comprehensive data. However, AI wearables are set to change this by continuously generating accurate and near real-time user health data.

These models use AI algorithms such as machine learning, deep learning, and neural networks to analyze data from fitness trackers. This can then predict potential future health conditions, from cardiovascular diseases to diabetes, based on a myriad of health parameters, allowing for early detection and preventative treatment.

10.3. Virtual Coaches and AI

Virtual coaching systems utilizing AI are growing in capability and sophistication. Unlike human trainers, they can offer 24/7 guidance, feedback, and health monitoring. They can also adapt workout plans according to your progress, schedule, or even mood.

Imagine having a personal coach in your ear during a workout, accurately analyzing your form, providing real-time feedback, and encouraging you when your motivation wanes.

10.4. Enhanced Biometric Monitoring

Biometric monitoring will also evolve to some truly advanced levels. We're already seeing fitness trackers that can monitor sleep, count steps, track calories, and measure heart rate. Next up, we might see technology capable of analyzing sweat composition for hydration and electrolyte balance, or devices monitoring blood glucose levels non-invasively, helping individuals manage conditions such as diabetes.

10.5. Emotional Health Tracking

While much emphasis has been placed on the integration of AI with physical health, there is potential for monitoring emotional health as well.

Algorithms could analyze user data such as cortisol levels, skin temperature, and sleep patterns to provide insights into their stress and emotional state. This could assist in providing recommendations for stress management techniques and harbor an overall well-being approach, further expanding the realm of fitness tracking.

10.6. Augmented Reality and Fitness

Apart from wearable technology, another exciting development is the fusion of AI, fitness tracking, and augmented reality. This could lead to highly immersive fitness experiences, like turning a routine workout into a virtual fitness adventure, which could increase adherence to fitness plans and ensure working out never feels like a chore.

Lastly, the open-source nature of AI development often means that with every advancement comes a wave of innovative applications from the global developer community, further enhancing what's possible in AI and fitness tracking.

Simply put, AI combined with fitness tracking devices is redefining the landscape of health and wellness, and the possibilities seem endless. It is these possibilities that invite us all to participate in shaping a future where fitness is not just attainable, but approachable, enjoyable, and deeply personalized.

Chapter 11. Wrap Up: Maximizing Your Fitness Goals with AI

As we move towards the conclusion of this comprehensive insight into AI-driven fitness technology, it's key to discuss and understand how we can truly take advantage of these new tools to attain our maximum fitness goals.

11.1. Embracing AI-Driven Personalization

In our journey through this guide, we have consistently seen how AI has brought about a unique level of personalization to fitness. These digitally calibrated tools can adjust to your individual body type, fitness level, overall goals, and even to the nuances of your mood and feelings. This means that instead of following a single, blanket approach, you now have tailor-fit routines and advice available to you on demand.

If you're just starting with a fitness regime, aim to take smaller steps initially. Let the AI apparatus know your current fitness status, your dietary habits, and preferred workout formats. Over time, as the system becomes accustomed to your needs and responses, it will help you increase the intensity of workouts, suggest healthier meal alternatives, and keep you motivated and accountable towards your goals.

11.2. Understanding the Data

One significant advantage of AI-driven fitness technologies is the wealth of data they collect and analyze. It's essential, however, to understand the basics of this data to fully exploit the benefits. For instance, knowing what your heart rate zones are and what they signify can help you optimize your training and recovery. Similarly, understanding how sleep data relates to recovery and muscle growth can help you plan your routine better.

Most of these tools come with a user-friendly dashboard that makes complex data easy to grasp. If there are terms or metrics you don't understand, don't hesitate to seek guidance. The more you comprehend the data, the better you'd be able to apply the insights.

11.3. Incorporating Tech into your Routine

At the core of it all, AI in fitness tracking is a tool—a powerful one, for sure, but a tool nonetheless. As with any tool, its effectiveness will largely depend on how we use it.

Begin by incorporating your AI-driven tech in your routine slowly. Use it to track your workouts, your heart rate, your sleep, and your nutrition. As you become accustomed to coordinating with the tool, you will start noticing trends and patterns. For example, you may notice you sleep better on the days you workout or your endurance improves as you incorporate more protein in your diet.

11.4. Ensuring Consistent Engagement

Consistency is key in any fitness journey, and the same is true when maximizing the benefits from your AI fitness tools. Ensure you are making consistent entries, whether it's logging your meals or marking your workouts. This gives the AI system a better understanding of your lifestyle and habits, thereby enabling it to make more accurate and personalized recommendations.

Engage with the tool as often as possible, make it a part of your daily routine and remember, these small regular entries could make a significant difference in your long term health goals.

11.5. Balancing Data with Intuition

While the data from your AI tools can provide incredible insights, it's essential to balance this information with your intuition and instinct. If your tool suggests pushing harder in your workout, but you feel overly fatigued, it's important to listen to your body and perhaps take it easy.

Similarly, ensure you are eating not just based on suggested calories but also considering your hunger and energy levels. Balancing data with intuition can help avoid burnout and keep your fitness journey enjoyable and sustainable.

11.6. Reflecting and Adjusting

Finally, take the time to reflect on the results and adjust as and when needed. Maybe a suggested diet plan is not working for you, or a suggested workout does not interest you. This is an iterative process, and learning from each cycle greatly enhances your journey.

Remember, fitness trackers, even AI-powered ones, are ultimately tools. They are there to assist and guide us. However, we're the ones leading the journey, and we have the power to tune, adjust, and redesign the route to best achieve our unique health goals.

By integrating these guidelines, we can smartly utilize the AI-enabled fitness trackers to take a calculated, data-driven, and effective leap towards enhanced wellness and fitness. This is only the beginning in the journey of AI in fitness tracking. As technology evolves, we can only predict that AI will keep on improving, offering us even more refined, personalized, and revolutionary ways to stay healthy and fit.